HEALING
OSTEOARTHRITIS
HANDS

EASY MEAL PLAN AND PAIN-FREE EXERCISES TO HEAL YOUR OWN THUMB, FINGERS AND WRIST.

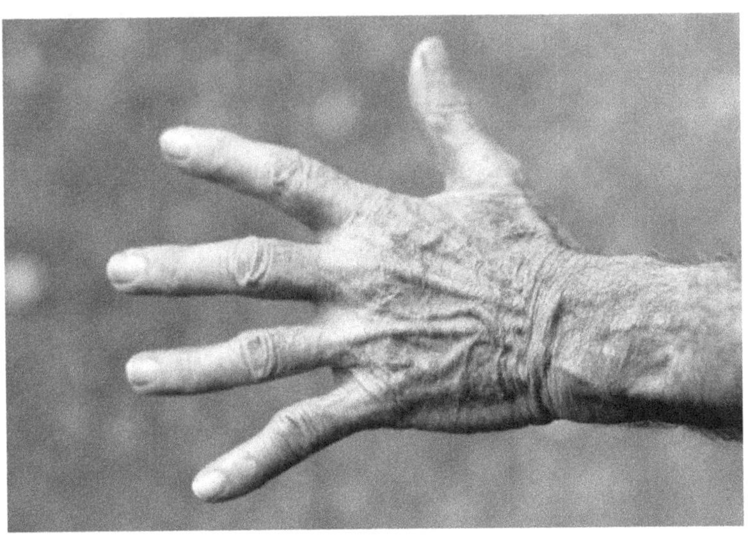

DR. KADEN WINTON

FREE EMAIL CONSULTATION

Dear Reader,

Thank you for choosing to embark on the healing journey with our book, ***"Healing Osteoarthritis Hands"*** Your support means the world to us, and we are deeply grateful for your trust.

As a token of our appreciation, we would like to offer you a unique opportunity. We are delighted to provide a complimentary email consultation where you`` can address any questions or challenges you may encounter while implementing the principles shared in our book.

Simply send me an email at wintonconsults@gmail.com and within 24 hours, you will receive a personalized response from me.

Please note that this free consultation offer is exclusively available to individuals who have purchased our book.

Once again, we extend our heartfelt thanks for your support, and we look forward to assisting you on your healing journey

Dedication

We dedicate this book to our beloved arthritis warriors, who have spent their days, months and years through pains. We are with you through this trying time of pain and agony, and we assure you that your pains won't linger for so long, because there is still hope to live a pain-free life.

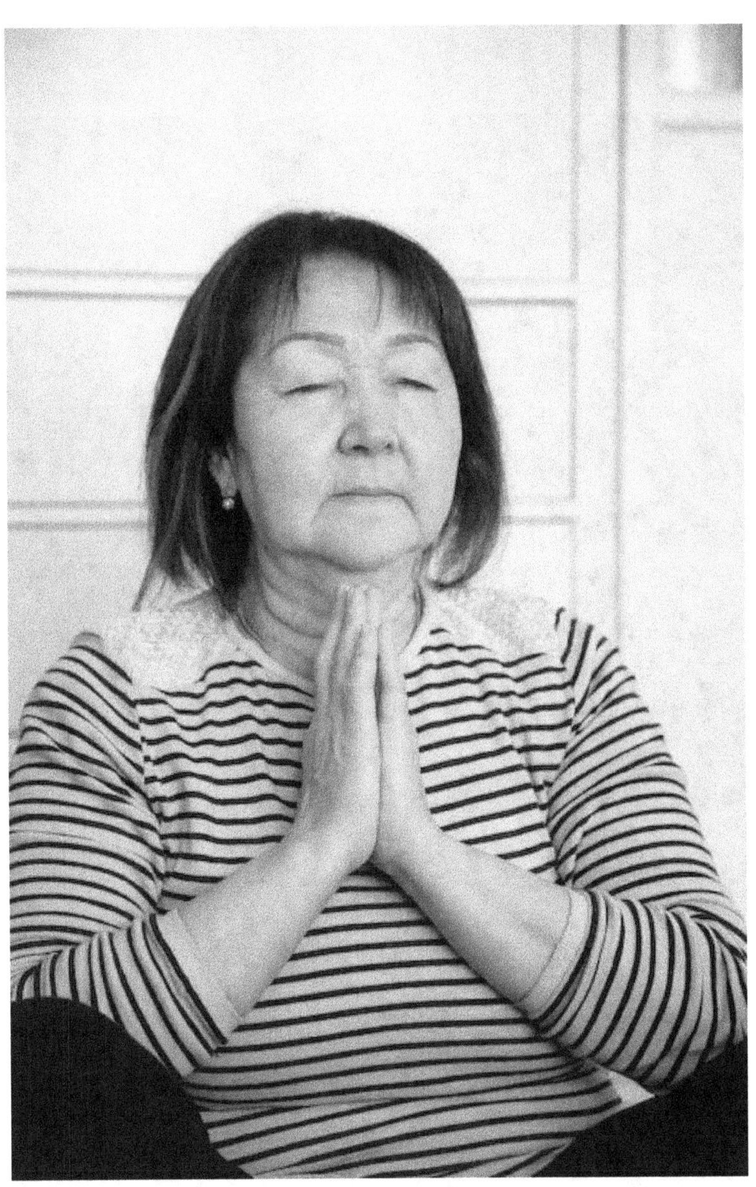

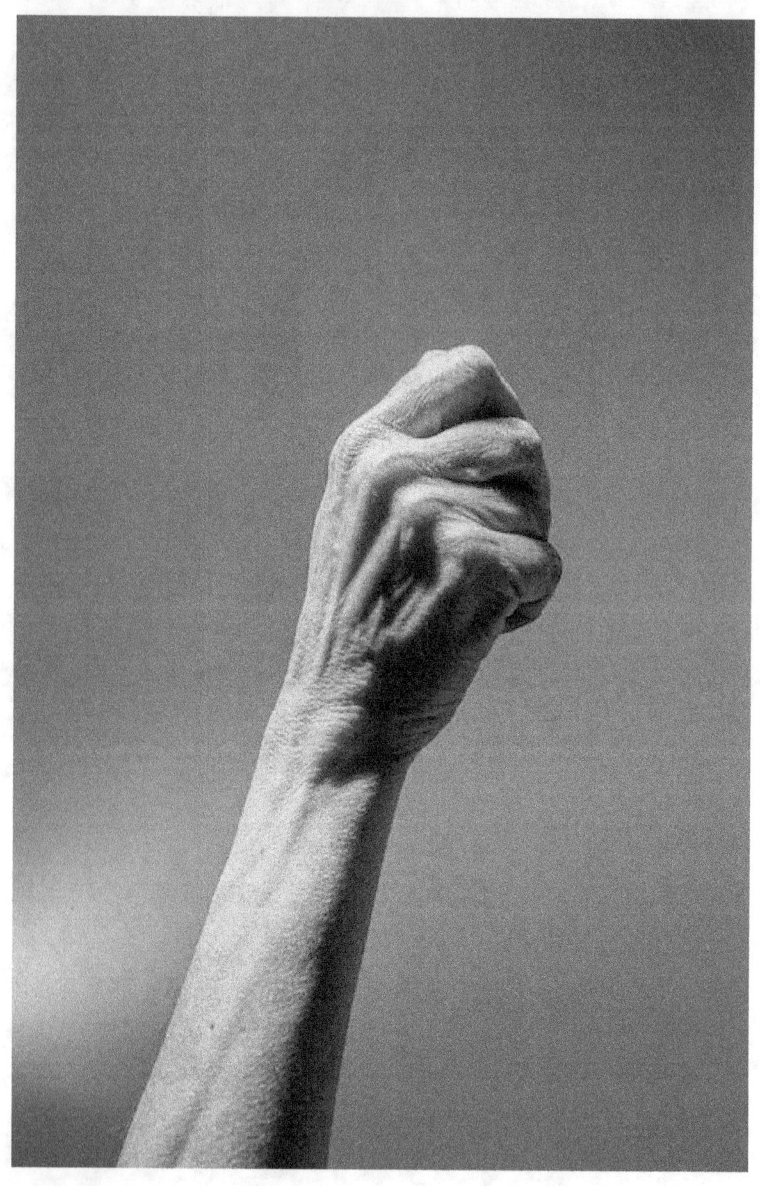

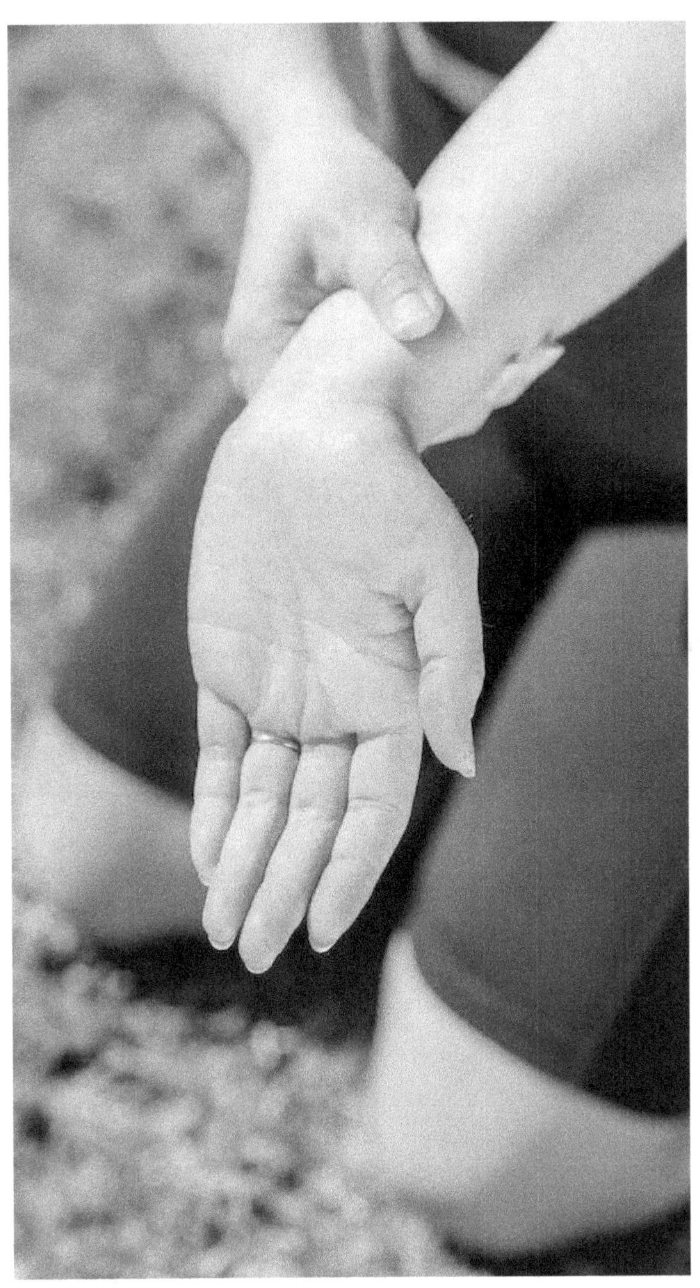

Table of Contents

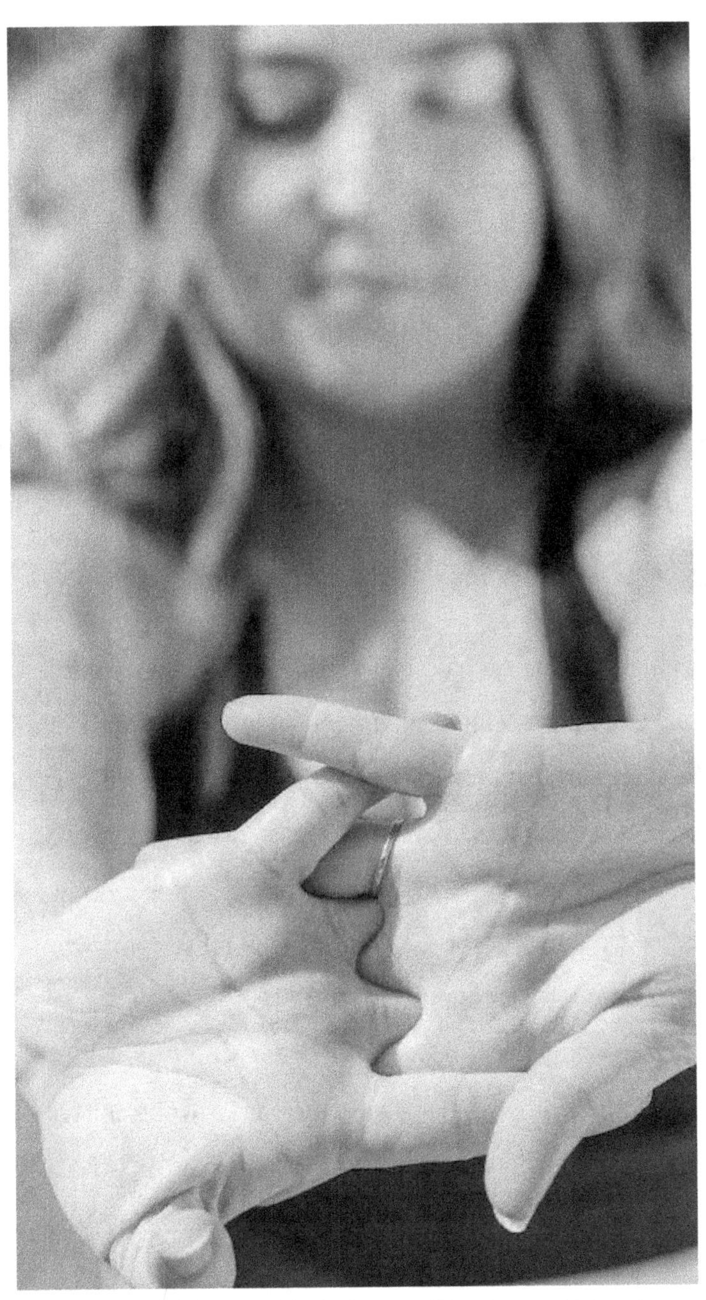

Introduction

In a quiet town, Sarah was a strong and resilient woman. She faced the loss of her beloved husband, leaving her with five beautiful children to raise. Despite being admired by many prominent men, Sarah remained focused on giving her kids the love and attention her late husband would have wanted for them.

Sarah got a job as a hairstylist in a small downtown salon to make ends meet. Her skilled hands and passion for braiding made her stand out among her colleagues, and her reputation spread far and wide. With her newfound success, Sarah could provide her children with what they needed, and she felt secure enough not to rely on financial support from the men who were continuously asking her out.

But fate had other plans. One day, Sarah woke up with an unusual pain in her right hand. She brushed it off at first, thinking it was from her work. But the pain persisted and worsened, making it hard for her to do simple tasks. The diagnosis confirmed her fears: she had osteoarthritis.

Sarah felt devastated, her hand health declined over time, and she had to opt for some painkillers, which provided little help; she felt relieved for a day or two, but it seems she is yet to tackle the root source of her predicaments, on the third day, the pain returned, this time more severe and Sarah had to stop working, thus, putting her family in financial trouble.

She couldn't provide as she used to for her kids, which was telling heavily as they grew thin and malnourished as the days ran by.

Just when hope seemed lost, her loyal customer and friend, Jane, noticed Sarah's absence from the salon and decided to come check up on her beloved stylist and friend. Tears rolled down Jane's eyes when she saw the present state of her friend, she comforted herself knowing she had faced similar challenges, and have a better treatment option to offer. Jane shared her husband's battle with osteoarthritis and offered hope with a special diet and exercise routine. Promising to bring the book that had helped her husband, Jane left, determined to help her friend.

Jane returned with the book the next day, and Sarah eagerly followed its guidance. She prepared anti-inflammatory meals and did gentle exercises. Gradually, she noticed an improvement in her condition. Though not completely healed after two weeks, Sarah didn't give up.

She continued with the book's recommendations. By the fifth week, she felt her strength returning, and her hands were almost pain-free. With gratitude, she got rehired in another salon and gradually earned enough money to provide for her children again.

Sarah never forgot the kindness of her friend Jane and the selfless support of Dr. Kaden Winton book, whose healing knowledge had given her a second chance at life. Her journey had been filled with hardships, but it also revealed the power of perseverance, friendship, and the healing potential found within the pages of a book.

Osteoarthritis is very common in the United States, affecting one out of every five people over 18. It is also the leading cause of disability in the United States. If osteoarthritis is not treated, the bones that make up the joint can lose their normal shape, making movement painful and significantly limiting the joint's range of motion. Though anyone can develop osteoarthritis, the risks increase significantly with age.

Osteoarthritis can affect any joint in the body, but it most commonly affects the hands, wrists, knees, and feet. The wrist, hand, and finger joints are among the most important joints for performing daily activities, which is why osteoarthritis is the most common type of arthritis.

How Do You Know If You Have Osteoarthritis?

Each type of osteoarthritis has its own set of symptoms, but there are some that are good general indicators of osteoarthritis development, such as:

• Pain or swelling in one or more joints

• Joints that appear red or feel warm to the touch

• Tender, stiff, or difficult-to-move joints

Hand osteoarthritis can be difficult to diagnose for a general practitioner because it can manifest in a variety of ways, and the symptoms can be difficult to recognize. The symptoms may appear and disappear over time. The pain could be mild and come on gradually, or it could come on quickly and cause intense, surging pain that goes away in a few hours. Alternatively, the symptoms could appear as something completely unrelated, such as fatigue or a rash. That is why it is critical to understand the warning signs and which symptoms indicate a more serious underlying problem. If you are experiencing any of the following symptoms, you should see a trained hand specialist.

• Three or more days of joint pain or stiffness

• Multiple episodes of red or joint warm over the course of a month

• Joint swelling

What Is The Treatment For Osteoarthritis?

When it comes to osteoarthritis treatment early diagnosis and detection is essential to developing a successful treatment and management plan for your joints. Treatment for osteoarthritis of the thumb, for example, differs from treatment for rheumatoid (RA), therefore it is very important you know the condition of your hand and how to go about it.

In this book we will be looking at basically two proven strategies for managing osteoarthritis; the dietary approach; that covers healthy eating of food with anti-inflammatory properties, and the exercise approach; which involves engaging in simple, yet effective hand exercises. As a bonus, we will as well incorporated some herbal remedies to help with the pain. So relax, grab some healthy juice and enjoy your read to wellness!

Can Osteoarthritis Be Prevented?

There are numerous things you can do in your daily life to reduce your chances of developing arthritis, including:

- Regular physical activity

- Maintaining a healthy weight

- Avoiding excessive repetitive movements

- Balancing activity with rest to avoid overworking the joints

- Maintaining a healthy immune system

These preventative methods are more effective depending on the location of your joint pain. If you have hand osteoarthritis, using hot and cold therapies may help relieve your pain. Furthermore, range-of-motion exercises can help maintain joint flexibility and prevent long-term stiffness.

These preventative measures will go a long way in helping you deal with the problem, if you suspect you have arthritis, consult your doctor or a specialist for a proper diagnosis.

In this book, we will primarily focus on two osteoarthritis management options that have proven to help patients with hand osteoarthritis live pain-free lives over the years. I would like you to read this book slowly and take your time to implement all which is revealed in this book. I am confident that in a short time, I will be hoping to see your healing testimonies.

Please contact us at wintonconsults@gmail.com if you encounter any difficulties while using our book. Good luck with your reading and healing!

Individuals who as feel arthritis pain in their knee can proceed to adopting this treatment plan.

Part One

Eating For Hand Arthritis

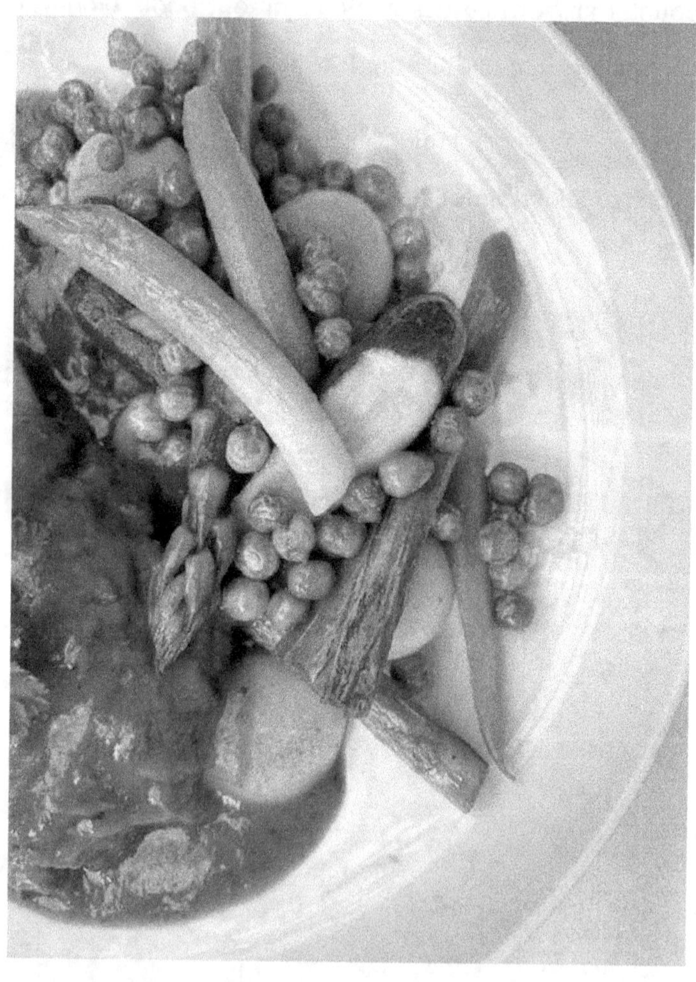

Chapter One

Is Your Diet Fighting Or Causing Your Pain?

FOOD IS OUR FUEL, just as gasoline is to a car. What we put into our bodies either moves us toward disease or towards health. Have you ever heard the expression, *"Which dog are you feeding?"* The *"dog"* who is fed will always win over the *"dog"* who is starved. The same is true for illness and pain. It will grow stronger if you feed it.

But who or what is the *"dog"* you're feeding? **INFLAMATION IS THE REAL CULPRIT.**

Inflammation is the root cause of almost all pain and disease, including joint pain! Pain is a signal from the body that something isn't working properly. And we become extremely motivated to alleviate that pain. BUT, rather than masking the pain with painkillers every few hours, we should focus on addressing the source of the pain. Or simply accept our fate. To address the root cause of joint pain, we must address the inflammatory process that has most likely been brewing beneath the body's surface for years.

You may be wondering where we got all of this inflammation. Our food is the primary source of inflammation. That means we can change the inflammatory processes with powerful nutrient products and food!

It's worth noting that, in addition to joint pain, chronic inflammation is a deadly side effect of both heart disease and cancer. Heart disease currently accounts for one in every four deaths, and the Centers for Disease Control (CDC) estimates that cancer kills 1,620 people every day in 2015.

What Are The Indicators That Hidden Inflammation Is Causing My Joint Pain?

• Having an inflammatory condition (such as osteoarthritis) and/or joint pain

• Reduced mobility (joints that do not "move well" and are stiff)

• Difficulty rising from a chair or getting out of bed

• Digestive issues (such as bloating or constipation)

• High cholesterol or heart disease • Sugar issues or diabetes

• Skin problems (such as rashes, hives, eczema, or psoriasis)

Do I Fight Or Feed Inflammation?

Some of these responses might surprise you! Here are some examples of lifestyle choices that contribute to inflammation:

• Consuming grains (pasta, bread, oatmeal, sandwiches, and crackers)

• Consuming sugar (fruit, stevia, honey, soda, jams, snacks, granola bars, and cookies)

• Regular dairy or yogurt consumption (which contains a type of sugar)

• Alcohol consumption (which causes inflammation)

• Inadequate sleeping habits

• High levels of stress

Here are some examples of anti-inflammatory lifestyle choices:

• Consuming leafy, dark greens on a daily basis (did you know that spinach has more calcium than milk!)

• Taking anti-inflammatory nutritional supplements (such as Vitamin D and Omega 3s).

• Stress-reduction techniques (such as meditation or yoga) to lower cortisol levels

• Increasing the use of "good fats" in the kitchen

• Avoiding processed foods

• Limiting consumption of non-organic or non-free range meats

How Can I Fight Joint Pain With Nutrition?

Your body is in an inflammatory state when you have arthritis. It is critical to consume foods that do not contribute to inflammation. What you eat may not cause inflammation, but it can put you at risk for other chronic diseases like diabetes, heart disease, and obesity. The following foods may cause more inflammation in your body:

Red meat: Red meat contains a high level of omega-6 fatty acid or saturated fat, which aggravates inflammation and pain, and contributes to obesity. Consuming a small amount of red meat can be beneficial because it provides nutrients such as iron. People with arthritis, on the other hand, may benefit from limiting themselves to one or two servings per week.

Sugary Drinks: Sugary drinks, such as coffee, can raise blood acidity, exacerbating inflammation. Reduce your intake of coffee and other sugary drinks in favor of more water, herbal tea, and fruit juice.

Sugar and Refined Flour: When you consume sugar, your blood sugar level can spike after eating simple carbohydrates that the body can easily break down. A spike in your blood sugar level causes your body to produce pro-inflammatory chemicals known as cytokines. Sugar can aggravate osteoarthritis symptoms, and inflammation can harm your joints. Sugar consumption can also cause weight gain and joint stress.

Fried Foods: Fried foods can aggravate inflammation. Cutting back on fried foods, on the other hand, can help reduce inflammation. Toxins in fried foods increase oxidation in the body's cells. These fattening foods contribute to obesity and aggravate arthritis.

Gluten: Gluten is a protein found in grains, including barley, wheat, and rye. All of these foods can contribute to the development of inflammation. If a person has celiac disease, eating gluten can trigger an immune response in the small intestine, resulting in bloating and diarrhea. In some cases, the inflammatory response can spread to the joints, exacerbating osteoarthritis symptoms.

Dairy Products: The type of protein found in dairy products can contribute to the development of osteoarthritis pain. The protein in this product may irritate the tissue around the joints in some cases.

Corn Oil: Many baked foods and snacks contain corn or oils high in omega-6 fatty acids. These snacks are highly satisfying to the taste buds, but they also cause inflammation.

Tobacco and Alcohol: Tobacco and alcohol use can cause a variety of health problems, some of which may affect the joints. People who smoke are more likely to develop rheumatoid arthritis, whereas people who drink alcohol are more likely to develop gout.

Processed foods: Processed foods require little cooking and contain preservatives that are high in ingredients that can cause inflammation. Processed foods are high in sugar, saturated fats, and refined flour, all of which are unhealthy and contribute to obesity.

Healthy Eating for Hands and Joint Health

Changing some of your daily eating habits can have a positive impact on your overall health. This is most likely something you already knew. Did you know that changing some of your daily foods can promote healthy joints and prevent joint conditions like hand arthritis? Everyone in today's world appears to believe that they can simply take pills for everything. While you can take pills, wouldn't you rather change your diet and go the natural route? There are many foods that can help prevent a variety of medical conditions. Here are some great foods for joint health.

Glucosamine

This substance occurs naturally in the body. This compound generates glycosaminoglycan, a molecule used in cartilage repair. So, if your cartilage is damaged, your body will begin to repair itself as long as you have enough glucosamine. The body's ability to produce glucosamine decreases with age. So you should do everything you can to help your body heal naturally. Glucosamine can be found in the following foods.

- Shrimp Shells

- Lobster Shells

- Crab Shells

- The majority of sports drinks

- Sweet Almond Oil

Manganese

This is a co-factor that aids in the formation of cartilage. Including manganese in your diet will help your body's glucosamine levels. Adding more manganese will accelerate and boost productivity. Manganese can be found in the following foods.

- Beans
- Whole Grain Breads
- Whole Grain Cereals
- Milk, Seafood
- Dark Leafy Vegetables
- Nuts

Omega-3 Fatty Acids

This can only be obtained through food or other supplements. This is not produced by your body. This means that if you do not include it in your diet, you will not have any in your system. These have anti-inflammatory properties that help with pain and swelling. When your joints become inflamed, they can cause excruciating pain. Instead of taking Motrin, try changing your diet. It can also help improve blood flow. The following foods are high in Omega 3 fatty acids.

- Salmon
- Cod
- cod liver oil
- flax seeds
- walnuts
- egg yolk
- Trout -Sardines

Vitamin C and E

Antioxidants like vitamin E works with Vitamin C to slow down the aging process. It improves and safeguards Vitamin C. These two vitamins are frequently found together in foods and work together in your body. If you don't have one, the other one can't do its job. So eating foods that are high in both vitamins is a good idea. Vitamin C, also known as the most well-known vitamin, aids in the formation of collagen in the body. Collagen is a protein found in bone, tendons, and cartilage. They also claim that it can help you live a longer life. The following foods are high in both vitamin C and vitamin E.

- Every Citrus Fruit
- Tomatoes
- Strawberries
- Cabbage
- Kiwi
- Potatoes
- Watermelon
- Broccoli
- Cantaloupe

- Papayas
- Corn
- Nuts
- Oats

These are just a few of the foods that promote joint health. Other ingredients found in foods for healthy joints include chondroitin, MSM, and silicon.

We understand that many people are tasked with preparing these meals as well as having a simple meal that meets their nutritional needs when it comes to managing arthritis. We have created a 7-day meal plan that will guide you through your healing journey.

I hope you are enjoying your read? Never hesitate to send us a mail @ wintonconsults@gmail.com should you have any challenge using our book. As an appreciation, we humbly ask you go give our book some ratings, your reviews will help us trim our future books to address your specific health challenges, thank you.

Chapter Two

Anti-inflammatory Food Prep Guide and Meal Plan for Hand Health

Incorporating some foods with antioxidant properties will go a long way in your healing journey, so you're far from the doctor's desk. Here's a detailed step-by-step meal preparation guide for anti-inflammatory breakfast, launch, dinner, snacks, smoothies and juice recipes required for your healing.

Meal Prep Guide - Anti-inflammatory breakfasts

Recipe 1: Overnight Turmeric Chia Pudding

Ingredients:

- 1/4 cup chia seeds

- 1 cup almond milk

- 1/2 teaspoon ground turmeric

- 1/2 teaspoon pure vanilla extract

- Fresh and chopped nuts for topping

Meal Prep

Step 1: In a container or jar with a tight-fitting lid, combine 1/4 cup chia seeds, 1 cup almond milk, 1/2 teaspoon ground turmeric, and 1/2 teaspoon vanilla extract

Step 2: Stir the mixture well to ensure that the chia seeds are evenly distributed and do not clump.

Step 3: Close the lid tightly and place the container in the refrigerator overnight or for at least 6 hours.

Step 4: In the morning, take the chia pudding out of the fridge and give it a good stir to break up any lumps.

Step 5: Place the chia pudding in a bowl and top with your favorite fresh berries and chopped nuts, adding flavor and texture.

Recipe 2: Vegan-Packed Egg Muffins

Ingredients:

- 6 large eggs

- 1/4 cup diced bell peppers

- 1/4 cup diced

- 1/4 cup chopped tomatoes

- 1/4 cup diced

- Salt and pepper to taste

Meal Prep

Step 1: Preheat your oven to 350°F (175°C) and lightly grease the muffin tin with spray or coconut oil.

Step 2: In a large mixing bowl, crack 6 large eggs and mix until well beaten.

Step 3: Add 1/4 cup each of the chopped peppers, spinach, tomatoes, and onion to the beaten eggs.

Step 4: Add salt and pepper to the mixture to taste and stir everything together until the vegetables are evenly distributed.

Step 5: Pour the egg and vegetable mixture into a greased muffin tin, filling each cup about 3/4 full.

Step 6: Bake the potato muffins in the preheated oven for 15-20 minutes or until completely set and lightly golden on top.

Step 7: Allow muffins to cool completely before transferring to an airtight container.

Step 8: Store the egg muffins in the fridge, and reheat them in the microwave or oven in the morning for a quick healthy breakfast.

Recipe 3: Green Smoothie Freezer Accessories

Ingredients

- 1 cup fresh spinach

- 1/2 ripe banana

- 1/2 cup pineapple pieces

- 1 teaspoon chia seeds

- 1 cup of orange juice

Meal Prep

Step 1: Prepare an individual freezer bag or container for each green smoothie.

Step 2: Add 1 cup fresh coconut, 1/2 ripe banana, 1/2 cup pineapple chunks, and 1 teaspoon chia seeds to each pack.

Step 3: Cover the bag or container tightly and store it in the fridge.

Step 4: In the morning, grab a green smoothie pack from the fridge and add the contents to the blender.

Step 5: Add 1 cup of orange juice to a blender and blend until smooth.

Step 6: Pour the green smoothie into a glass for a healthy and nutrient-dense breakfast.

Recipe 4: Smoked avocado and salmon toast

Ingredients:

- 2 slices of whole grain bread (gluten-free if desired).

- 1 sliced avocado

- Smoked salmon slices

- Fresh fennel and lemon garnish

Meal Prep

Step 1: Cut 2 slices of bread and place them in a resalable bag or container.

Step 2: In a separate bowl, mash the cooked avocado and add strained lemon juice to prevent browning.

Step 3: Store sliced avocado and lemon zest in the refrigerator.

Step 4 Toast the bread slices in the morning until golden and crispy.

Step 5: Sprinkle the sliced avocado on the breadcrumbs and top with the smoked salmon.

Step 6: Garnish with fennel and fresh lemon zest for flavor and presentation.

By following this step-by-step meal preparation guide, you can easily and easily have a week's worth of delicious antioxidant breakfasts. This breakfast fix will help support your journey towards healing osteoarthritis in your hands while starting your day in a healthy way. Happy meal prepping!

Meal Prep Guide - Anti-inflammatory Lunches

Lunchtime calls for a healthy and satisfying meal that provides your body with essential nutrients and reduces inflammation. Prepare this anti-inflammatory lunch in advance for a fun week of lunches.

Recipe 1: Grilled Salmon Salad

Ingredients:

- Grilled salmon fillet

- A mixture of green

- Cherry tomatoes

- A cut-out bowl

- The snowflake

- Olive oil and lemon juice

Meal Prep

Step 1: Heat salmon and cool until evenly cooked.

Step 2: Place mixed vegetables, cherry tomatoes, sliced cucumber, and sliced avocado in individual airtight bowls.

Step 3: Top the salad with the fried salmon fillet.

Step 4: Drizzle the salad with olive oil and lemon zest, or save the dressing in a separate container for later pouring.

Step 5: Cover the jars and refrigerate until ready to eat. Enjoy a fresh and anti-inflammatory salmon salad for lunch.

Recipe 2: Quinoa stuffing

Ingredients:

- Bell pepper (any color).

- cooked quinoa

-Stir in spinach and mushrooms

- Sliced tomatoes

Meal Prep

Step 1: Cut off the tops of the bell peppers and remove the seeds and membrane.

Step 2: In a mixing bowl, combine the cooked quinoa, ground spinach, mushrooms, and diced tomatoes.

Step 3: Fill the hollow shells with the quinoa mixture.

Step 4: Transfer the egg yolks to an airtight container.

Step 5: After eating, microwave the potato stuffing until fully heated. Enjoy a delicious anti-inflammatory lunch.

Recipe 3: Chutney and Vegetable Garnish

Ingredients:

- Cooked sauce

- Mixed (broccoli, bell peppers, carrots).

-Twist (low sodium soy sauce, garlic, ginger).

- Brown Rice (Optional).

Meal Prep:

Step 1: Stir the vegetable mixture until soft and crispy in a saucepan or wok.

Step 2: Add the cooked sauce to the pan and pour the stir-sauce over the mixture.

Step 3: Stir everything together until the sauce and vegetables are covered in the sauce.

Step 4: Divide sauce and vegetable stir-fry among individual food prep containers.

Step 5: Serve over brown rice of your choice or store the rice separately for later pairing. Refrigerate until lunchtime.

Recipe 4: Lentils & Vegetable Soup

Ingredients:

- Red Lentils

- chopped Carrots, celery and onion

- Vegetable Broth

- Turmeric and cumin, respectively for flavor

Meal Prep

Step 1: In a pot, combine red lentils, shredded carrots, celery, onions, and vegetable broth.

Step 2: Season the soup with turmeric and cumin for flavor and anti-inflammatory benefits.

Step 3: Bring the soup to a simmer, then reduce the heat and simmer until the corn and vegetables are tender.

Step 4: Allow the soup to cool slightly before transferring to individual airtight containers.

Step 5: Refrigerate the dishes until lunchtime. Reheat lentil and vegetable soup for a comforting and nutritious lunch.

Following this meal preparation guide will prepare you for a week's worth of anti-inflammatory lunches. These lunch options will not only keep you entertained but will help your quest for osteoarthritis solutions at hand. Enjoy!

Meal Prep Guide - Anti-Inflammatory Dinner

Start your day with a delicious and anti-inflammatory dinner that nourishes your body and soothes inflammation. This meal prep idea will save you time in the kitchen and ensure you have healthy dinners throughout the week.

Recipe 1: Baked Turmeric Chicken

Ingredients

- Boneless, skinless chicken breast

- Turmeric, paprika, and garlic powder

Meal Prep

Step 1: Preheat your oven to 375°F (190°C) and line a baking sheet with parchment paper.

Step 2: Mix the chicken breasts with turmeric seasoning, paprika, and garlic powder.

Step 3: Place the stuffed chicken breasts on the prepared baking sheet.

Step 4: Roast the chicken in the preheated oven for 25-30 minutes or until cooked through and not pink in the center.

Step 5: Allow the chicken to cool before storing it in individual food storage containers.

Step 6: When it's time for dinner, put the dishes in the fridge for easy reheating.

Recipe 2: Quinoa and kale salad

Ingredients:

- Cooked quinoa

- Massaged Kale

- Dried cranberries

- Roasted almonds

- Garnish with lemon-tahini

Meal Prep

Step 1: Combine the cooked quinoa and marinated kale in a large mixing bowl.

Step 2: Add dried cranberries and ground almonds to taste and smooth.

Step 3: Drizzle the lemon tahini dressing over the salad for a creamy and tangy finish.

Step 4 Toss everything together until the ingredients are evenly distributed.

Step 5: Divide the quinoa and kale salad into storage containers and refrigerate for later use.

Recipe 3: Potato and black bean tacos

Ingredients:

  - The sliced slices

  - The black hole

  - The snowflake

  - The Salsa Verde

  - Corn tortillas

Meal Prep

Step 1: Prepare the mashed potatoes by cutting them into bite-sized pieces and searing them in the oven.

Step 2: Reserve the cooked black beans and sliced avocado in a separate bowl.

Step 3: Place salsa verde in a small bowl and serve.

Step 4: Heat corn tortillas, fill them with mashed potatoes, black beans, and avocado slices, and assemble the tacos.

Step 5: Top the tacos with salsa verde for a delicious and healthy dinner.

Recipe 4: Ginger-Turmeric Veggie Stir-Fry

Ingredients:

- A variety of vegetables (broccoli, bell peppers, snap peas).

- Crushed tofu or tempeh

- Add ginger turmeric Sauce

- Brown Rice

Meal Prep

Step 1: In a saucepan or wok, stir various vegetables until soft and crispy.

Step 2: Add the chopped tofu or tempeh to the pan and pour the ginger and turmeric sauce over the mixture.

Step 3: Stir everything together until the vegetables are coated with the fragrant tofu or tempeh.

Step 4: Stir-fry over brown rice for a healthy and satisfying dinner.

Step 5: Alternatively, keep the stir-fry and brown rice separately for meal prep and combine when ready to eat.

If you follow this meal preparation guide, you'll have a week's worth of antibacterial dinners at your fingertips. These dinner options will satisfy you and help your journey to healing hand arthritis. Have a stress-free and healthy dinner every night!

Meal Prep Guide - Antioxidant Snacks

Keep your energy constant throughout the day with these delicious and antioxidant snacks. Preparing these snacks in advance gives you healthy options whenever you are hungry.

Recipe 1: Greek Yogurt Parfait

Ingredients:

- Greek yogurt

- Fresh (blueberries, strawberries, or raspberries).

- Honey or maple syrup

- almonds or walnuts (optional).

Meal Prep

Step 1: Place Greek yogurt and fresh fruit in small airtight containers or bowls.

Step 2: Drizzle the curd berries with honey or maple syrup for natural sweetness.

Step 3: Add some chopped almonds or walnuts for added crunch and nutrition.

Step 4: Lid the jars and refrigerate the parfaits for a quick and satisfying meal.

Recipe 2: Veggie sticks with hummus

Ingredients:

- The carrot sticks

- Cucumber slices

- Flakes of bell pepper

- Cherry tomatoes

- Hummus for dipping

Meal Prep

Step 1: Wash and chop carrot sticks, cucumber slices, bell pepper flakes, and cherry tomatoes.

Step 2: Place the veggie sticks in a bowl, and add a generous serving of hummus for dipping.

Step 3: Close the jars and store them in the fridge for a crisp and nutritious meal.

Recipe 3: Energy-boosting Trial Mix

Ingredients:

- Raw Almonds

- Pumpkin seeds

- Dried cranberries

- Unsweetened coconut flakes

- Dark Chocolate Chips (optional).

Meal Prep

Step 1: In a large mixing bowl, combine raw almonds, coconut seeds, dried cranberries, and unsweetened coconut milk.

Step 2: Alternatively, add some dark chocolate for a bit of fun.

Step 3: Toss everything together until the ingredients are evenly distributed.

Step 4: Partition the trial Mix in individual bottles or jars for easy pick-up and go.

Recipes 4: Rice Cake with Avocado and Radish

Ingredients:

- Rice cake

- Sliced avocado

- Chopped radishes

- Fresh lemon juice

- Sea salt and black pepper

Meal Prep

Step 1: Mash the ripe avocado in a bowl and add freshly squeezed lemon juice to make it sticky.

Step 2: Spread the avocado mixture over the rice cakes to create a satisfying base.

Step 3: Add thinly sliced radishes, sea salt, and black pepper to the rice cake to make it nice and soft.

Step 4: Store the avocado rice cake in an airtight container for a quick healthy meal.

By preparing these antioxidant foods in advance, you can satisfy your cravings with healthy ingredients that support your journey to osteoarthritis prevention in your hands. Enjoy these delicious and simple snacks throughout the day!

Prep Guide - Antibacterial Juice

Hydrate and rejuvenate your body with this nourishing and antioxidant juice. By prepping this juice ahead of time, you can enjoy daily doses of vitamins and antioxidants to support your health and overall healing journey.

Recipe 1: Turmeric Extract

Ingredients:

- Orange

- The carrots

- Fresh turmeric

- Fresh ginger

Prep

Step 1: Peel and slice the coconut.

Step 2: Wash and thinly slice the carrots.

Step 3: Remove fresh turmeric root and nut-sized pieces of fresh ginger.

Step 4: Put all the ingredients through a juicer and extract warm, immune-boosting water.

Step 5: Pour the juice into individual airtight containers and store it in the fridge.

Step 6: Shake well before drinking and savor the zesty and anti-inflammatory goodness.

Recipe 2: Green Anti-Inflammatory Elixir

Ingredients:

- Cucumber

- Celery

- Black paper

- Fresh lemon juice

- Fresh Parsley

Prep

Step 1: Wash and slice cucumber and celery.

Step 2: Chop the banana leaves into small pieces.

Step 3: Soak whole fresh lemons in water.

Step 4: Add a handful of fresh parsley for nutrition and flavor.

Step 5: Put all the ingredients through a juicer to get the vibrant green elixir.

Step 6: Pour the juice into individual airtight containers and refrigerate until enjoyed.

Recipe 3: Pineapple Ginger Juice

Ingredients:

- Fresh pineapple chunks

- Fresh ginger

- Mint leaves (optional).

- Coconut water

Prep

Step 1: Peel and slice fresh pineapple.

Step 2: Remove a nut-sized chunk of fresh ginger.

Step 3: Rinse and add fresh mint leaves for a fresh burst.

Step 4: Combine all ingredients in a blender or juicer and blend until smooth.

Step 5: Clean the water and remove any lines.

Step 6: Pour the pineapple ginger juice into individual jars and store it in the fridge.

Recipe 4: Anti-inflammatory berry

Ingredients:

- Mixed fruits (blueberries, strawberries, raspberries).

- Fresh lemon juice

- Water or coconut water

Prep

Step 1: Wash the fruit mixture thoroughly.

Step 2: Add fresh lemon juice and turn sharp.

Step 3: Combine fruit and lemon juice in a blender or juicer.

Step 4: Add water or orange juice to achieve desired results.

Step 5: Blend until smooth, skimming if necessary.

Step 6: Store the berry anti-inflammatory tonic in individual airtight containers for a refreshing and healthy drink.

By incorporating these antioxidants into your diet plan, you can up your hydration game and reap the benefits of a healthy body. Cheers to a healthier and much more vibrant you!

Prep Guide - Anti-Inflammatory Smoothies

Create a quick and satisfying way to support your hand health and healing with these delicious and nutrient-dense smoothies. Preparing these smoothies beforehand gives you extra nutrients ready to go whenever you need to grab them.

Recipe 1: *Tropical Turmeric Smoothie*

Ingredients:

- Pineapple slices

- Sliced mango pieces

- Fresh turmeric

- Fresh ginger

- Coconut milk or almond milk

Prep

Step 1: Remove fresh turmeric root and fresh ginger peel and chop.

Step 2: In a blender, combine frozen pineapple pieces, frozen mango pieces, turmeric, and ginger.

Step 3: Add coconut or almond milk to the blender to create a creamy and warm mixture.

Step 4: Blend until smooth and creamy, adjusting the amount of milk to your liking.

Step 5: Pour the smoothie into individual airtight containers and refrigerate until ready to enjoy.

Recipes 2: *Berry Avocado Happy Smoothie*

Ingredients:

- Mixed fruits (blueberries, strawberries, raspberries).

- Sliced avocado

- Fresh spinach or banana leaves

- Greek Yogurt (Optional).

- Water or coconut water

Prep

Step 1: Wash the mixed greens and the fresh spinach or kale leaves.

Step 2: Slice the ripe avocado and remove the flesh.

Step 3: In a blender, combine the mixed fruit, avocado, and fresh vegetables.

Step 4: Add a dollop of Greek yogurt for extra creaminess (if desired).

Step 5: Pour water or orange juice into the blender to achieve desired consistency.

Step 6: Blend the smoothie until smooth and pour the smoothie into individual bowls for storage.

Recipe 3: *Ginger-Beet Antioxidant Smoothie*

Ingredients:

- Boiled and dried beets (cold).

- Fresh ginger

- Fresh orange juice

- Fresh lime juice

- Honey or maple syrup (optional)

Prep

Step 1: Peel and chop fresh ginger.

Step 2: In a blender, combine cooked, peeled beets and fresh ginger.

Step 3: Squeeze orange and fresh lime juice for a zesty punch.

Step 4: If desired, add honey or maple syrup for a little sweetness.

Step 5: Blend until the ingredients are well incorporated, and the smoothie is velvety.

Step 6: Place the ginger-beet antioxidant smoothie in individual airtight containers and refrigerate.

Recipe 4: Creamy Almond Butter Banana Smoothie

Ingredients:

- Ripe bananas

- Almond butter

- Rolled oats

- Cinnamon

- Almond milk or soy milk

Prep

Step 1: Peel the ripe banana and divide it into pieces.

Step 2: Combine the banana slices with a tablespoon of almond butter and a handful of rolled oats in a blender.

Step 3: Add a few drops of cinnamon for a warm, comforting taste.

Step 4: Pour almond or soy milk into a blender to achieve the desired consistency.

Step 5: Blend until all the ingredients are well combined and have a creamy almond butter banana smoothie.

Step 6: Store smoothies in individual airtight containers and refrigerate until ready to enjoy.

You can easily incorporate more nutrition and health benefits into your daily routine by preparing these antioxidant smoothies in advance. Enjoy these velvety and delicious smoothies as part of your journey to heal osteoarthritis in your hands. Cheers to vibrant health and sweet bud satisfaction!

As guides, we created a 7-day meal plan to help you with your choices on this healing trip;

Day 1:

- Breakfast: Overnight turmeric chia pudding

- Lunch: Grilled salmon salad

- Dinner: Baked Turmeric Chicken

- Snacks: Greek Yogurt Parfait

- Juice: Citrusy Turmeric juice

Day 2:

- Breakfast: Vegan-packed egg muffins

- Lunch: Quinoa with bell peppers

- Dinner: Quinoa and kale salad

- Snack: Veggie sticks with hummus

- Smoothies: Tropical turmeric smoothies

Day 3:

- Breakfast: Green Smoothie Freezer Pack

- Lunch: Chickpea and vegetable soup

- Dinner: Sweet potato and black bean tacos

- Snack: Energy-boosting trail mix

- Juice: Green anti-inflammatory Elixir

Day 4:

- Breakfast: Smoked avocado and salmon toast

- Lunch: Lentil and vegetable soup

- Dinner: Ginger-turmeric veggie Stir-Fry

- Snack: Rice cake with avocado and radish

- Smoothie: Berry Avocado Happy Smoothie

Day 5:

- Breakfast: Finger Squeezes

- Lunch: Greek Yogurt Parfait

- Dinner: Pineapple Ginger Elixir

- Diet: Mixed Berry Antioxidant Smoothie

- Juice: Berry anti-inflammatory Tonic

Day 6:

- Breakfast: Thumbs up

- Lunch: Veggie sticks with hummus

- Dinner: Creamy almond butter kale smoothie

- Snack: Energy-boosting trail mix

- Smoothie: Ginger-Beet Antioxidant Smoothie

Day 7:

- Breakfast: Fist Openings

- Lunch: Quinoa and kale salad

- Dinner: Green anti-inflammatory elixir

- Snack: Rice cake with avocado and radish

- Juice: Tropical Turmeric Smoothie

Note: Ensure you drink plenty of water throughout the day to stay well-hydrated and support your body's natural healing process. Feel free to adjust the size and materials of the accessories based on your personal needs and preferences. Enjoy this delicious and healthy 7-day meal plan to promote anti-inflammatory benefits and support your journey towards healing osteoarthritis in your hands. Enjoy!

Anti-inflammatory Meal plan Grocery list

Starting an anti-inflammatory diet plan can have many health benefits, as well as many challenges; such as knowing the right food list to buy from the grocery shop.

To ensure an easy shopping experience, we have created a customized shopping list that included all the essential elements of the 7-Day Diet Plan, thus making your meal prep an easy one.

Proteins:

- Boneless, skinless chicken breast

- Salmon fillets

- Tofu or tempeh

- Eggs

- Greek yogurt

Grain:

- The Quinoa

- The blue sky

- Bottled oats

Vegetables:

- A mixture of green

- Cherry tomatoes

- Cucumber

- Avocado

- Bell peppers (various colors).

- Carrots

- Celery

- Spinach or Kale leaves

- The snowflake

- Red lentils

- Beets

- Radishes

Fruits:

- Orange

- Lemon

- Lime

- Pineapple

- Mango

- Fruits (blueberries, strawberries, raspberries).

Nuts and Seeds:

- Raw almonds

- Pumpkin seeds

- Dried cranberries

- Chopped almonds or walnuts

Herbs & Spices:

- Turmeric powder

- Paprika

- Garlic powder

- Cumin seeds

- Cinnamon

- Fresh turmeric root

- Fresh ginger

- Fresh mint leaves

- Fresh parsley

Milk and Substitutes:

- Coconut milk

- Almond milk

- Hummus

Spices and Condiments:

- Olive oil

- Honey or maple syrup

- Low sodium soy sauce

- The Salsa Verde

- Lemon–tahini dressing

Bakery & Deli:

- Rice cake

- Corn tortillas

Variety:

- Chia seeds

- Coconut

- Dark Chocolate Chips (optional).

- Water or coconut water

With this comprehensive shopping list, you'll have everything you need to embark on a week-long journey of nutrition and healing. Get ready to enjoy some fun anti-inflammatory foods that not only support your hand health but your overall recovery as well.

Join us in Part 2 as we explore advanced medicine, combining the power of exercise and nutrition to strengthen your hands and promote a vibrant, pain-free life.

I hope you are enjoying your read? Never hesitate to send us a mail @ wintonconsults@gmail.com should you have any challenge using our book. As an appreciation, we humbly ask you go give our book some ratings, your reviews will help us trim our future books to address your specific health challenges, thank you.

Pain- Free Osteoarthritis Hand Exercises

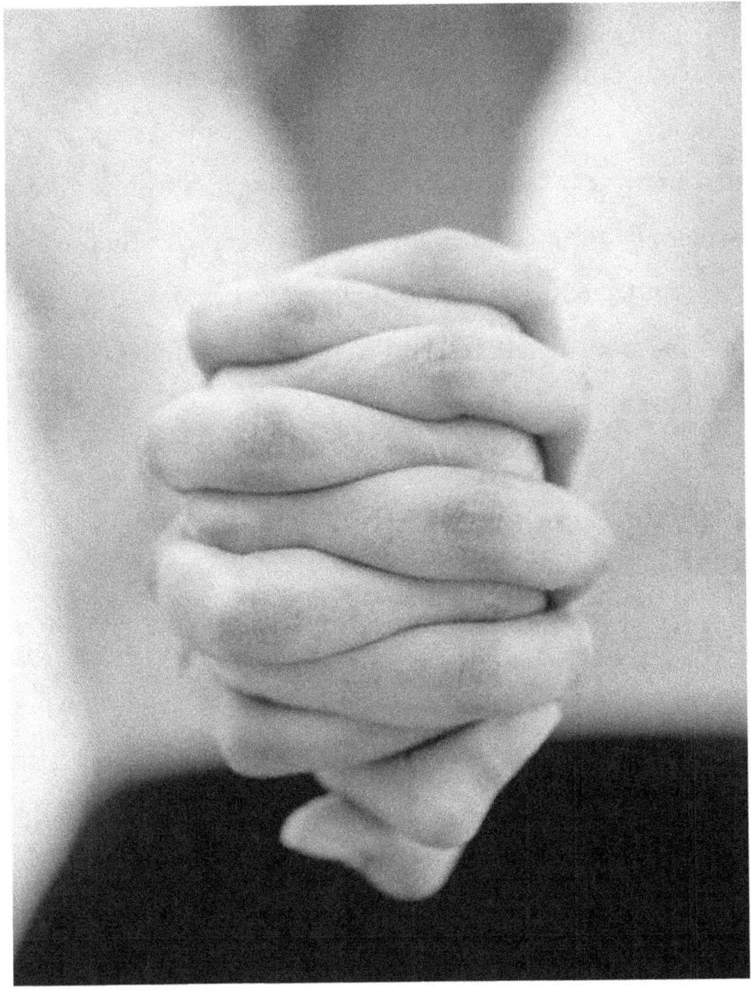

Chapter Two

What Exercises Works?

Welcome to hand exercises for osteoarthritis, where simplicity meets efficacy. This comprehensive guide delves into improving hand mobility and alleviating osteoarthritis symptoms through carefully crafted exercises. Tailored to target affected areas, these routines foster joint flexibility and muscle strength, empowering you on your journey to hand health.

Unraveling the Mechanisms of Action for Hand Exercise

Over the years a lot of people continue to ask the big question; how do these seemingly simple exercises work wonders for your hands? However, as they engage more with these seemingly simple exercise, they begin to unravel the healing mechanisms that lie beneath the surface:

1. Joint Lubrication and Nutrition:

These simple yet effective exercises, trigger the stimulation of synovial fluid production. This natural lubricant gracefully circulates within the hand joints, nurturing cartilage and minimizing friction. Behold improved joint lubrication, gracefully enhancing mobility while banishing osteoarthritis discomfort.

2. Strengthening Muscles and Tendons:

These simple yet effective exercises, embraces the power of targeted hand and forearm movements, thus, fortifying and supporting muscles and tendons. This amplified strength bestows greater stability upon your hands, unburdening affected areas and fostering smoother daily movements.

3. Enhancing Range of Motion:

These exercises promotes supple movement in the fingers and wrists, thus, preventing stiffness and improve the ability to perform daily tasks with ease.

4. Promoting Blood Flow and Circulation:

These simple, yet effective exercises increases blood flow to the hands, ensuring a steady supply of essential nutrients and oxygen to the joints. This blood circulation aids in repairing tissues, reducing inflammation, and contributing to overall hand health.

5. Pain Management and Endorphin Release:

This simple, yet effective exercise triggers the release of endorphins, the body's natural pain relievers. These endorphins not only alleviate arthritis-related discomfort but also have a positive impact on emotional well-being.

Props Needed To Start Your Exercise:

As you immerse yourself in these exercises, acquaint yourself with the captivating range of props that enhance your hand exercise routine:

1. Therapeutic Hand Putty or Stress Balls

2. Resistance Bands

3. Finger Extensors and Flexors

4. Finger Massagers

5. Grip Strengtheners

Safety Guidelines

To get the most out of hand exercises, you should consider the following guidelines.

1. **Consult with a health care professional:**

Seek the guidance of a certified health professional or hand therapist before beginning any exercise program. Individualized recommendations ensure that exercise is safe and tailored to individual needs.

2. **Start sequence:** Start with gentle exercises and gradually increase the intensity and duration over time. This allows the arm to rotate to move freely.

3. **Listen to your body:** Pay close attention to how your hands feel during and after exercise. If any pain or discomfort arises, change the exercise or take a break.

4. **Heating and cooling:** Before exercising, do a gentle warm-up to condition your arm muscles and then perform cooling exercises to relax.

5. **Consistency is key:** Regular exercise, preferably three to four times a week, is essential to improve hand movement and function.

Osteoarthritis Hand, Fingers, and Thumb Exercises

Exercise 1: Finger Squeezes

Let's explore finger squeezes, a simple yet effective exercise for stronger, more flexible hands. Follow these steps to improve your grip and dexterity.

Instructions:

1. Extend your fingers fully, like a painter's brush on a canvas.

2. Gently curl your fingers into a fist, holding for a few seconds.

3. Slowly release and return to the extended position.

4. Repeat the squeezing motion 10 to 15 times.

Tips:

- Perform the exercise slowly and focus on the sensations in your fingers and hands.

- Keep your wrist in a comfortable position.

- If you feel any pain, reduce the intensity of the squeeze or consult a healthcare professional.

Include finger squeezes in your daily routine to maintain hand strength, especially if you have osteoarthritis. Regular practice will make everyday tasks easier and more comfortable.

Exercise 2: Thumb Touches

Thumb touches are great for enhancing thumb mobility and coordination. Let's begin this beneficial exercise.

Instructions:

1. Start with your hand open and your fingers extended.

2. Gently bring your thumb toward the base of your pinky finger.

3. Hold for a moment, feeling the stretch in your thumb.

4. Release and repeat with each finger's base (index, middle, ring, and pinky).

Tips:

- Perform the motion slowly and mindfully.

- Keep your fingers extended and your wrist relaxed.

- If there's any discomfort, adjust the range of motion or consult a healthcare professional.

Include thumb touches in your daily routine to maintain flexibility and improve fine motor skills, especially if you have osteoarthritis in the thumb. This exercise can help alleviate discomfort and enhance overall thumb function.

Exercise 3: Fist Openings

Fist openings offer a gentle yet effective exercise for your hand and wrist muscles. Let's work on flexibility and reduce stiffness together.

Instructions:

1. Start with your hand relaxed and open.

2. Slowly curl your fingers inward to form a gentle fist.

3. Hold the fist for a few seconds, feeling the stretch.

4. Gradually release your fingers, opening your hand.

Tips:

- Perform the exercise smoothly and with control.

- Keep your wrist in a neutral position to avoid strain.

- If you feel any discomfort, adjust the fist formation or consult a healthcare professional.

Include fist openings in your daily hand exercise routine to maintain flexibility and reduce stiffness. This exercise can be particularly helpful in easing arthritis-related discomfort and enhancing hand function for various daily tasks.

Exercise 4: Wrist Flexor Stretch

The wrist flexor stretch targets wrist and forearm muscles to improve flexibility and relieve Tension. Let's get started.

Instructions:

1. Extend your arm in front of you, palm facing down.

2. Use your other hand to gently bend your wrist, pulling your fingers slightly towards your body.

3. Feel the stretch in your forearm and wrist.

4. Hold for 15-30 seconds, breathing deeply.

5. Release and repeat, on the other hand.

Tips:

- Keep your fingers relaxed during the stretch.

- Avoid overstretching and stay within a comfortable range.

- If you feel any pain, adjust the intensity or consult a healthcare professional.

Incorporating the wrist flexor stretches into your daily routine can help maintain wrist flexibility and relieve forearm tension. This exercise is an excellent addition to managing hand arthritis, providing relief and enhancing overall wrist function.

Exercise 5: Wrist Extensor Stretch

The wrist extensor stretch targets wrist and forearm muscles to improve flexibility and reduce stiffness. Let's give it a try.

Instructions:

1. Start with your arm extended in front of you, palm facing up.

2. Use your other hand to gently bend your wrist, pulling your fingers slightly downwards.

3. Feel the stretch on the top side of your forearm and wrist.

4. Hold for 15-30 seconds, breathing deeply.

5. Release and repeat, on the other hand.

Tips:

- Keep your fingers and hand relaxed during the stretch.

- Stay within a comfortable range and avoid overstretching.

- If you experience discomfort, adjust the intensity or consult a healthcare professional.

Incorporating the wrist extensor stretch into your daily routine can help maintain wrist flexibility and relieve forearm tension. This exercise is a great addition to managing hand arthritis, providing relief, and enhancing overall wrist function. Keep embracing these exercises to nurture the health of your hands and empower yourself on your journey to well-being.

I hope you are enjoying your read? Never hesitate to send us a mail @ winantonconsults@gmail.com should you have any challenge using our book. As an appreciation, we humbly ask you go give our book some ratings, your reviews will help us trim our future books to address your specific health challenges, thank you.

Get ready to strengthen those fingers and enhance hand mobility with a set of easy yet potent exercises! Let's dive into the world of finger taps and thumb circles, designed to boost your finger strength and flexibility.

Exercise 6: Finger Taps

Finger taps are a breeze! Just stretch those fingers comfortably and tap each separately on a firm surface, like a trusty table. Keep it steady and smooth. Don't forget to reverse the order and tap them back in the opposite direction. Let the rhythm flow for 15-30 seconds or more if you're comfy.

Tips:

- Stay cool and relaxed while tapping; no need to tense up those fingers.

- Keep the pace even and steady for all the fingers.

- If any discomfort creeps in, tone down the intensity or see a healthcare pro.

Go ahead and incorporate fingertips into your daily routine. Your fingers will thank you for improved strength and coordination, perfect for handling everyday tasks with ease. Great for managing osteoarthritis too!

Exercise 7: Thumb Circles

Hey there, thumbs up for thumb circles! Just stretch that hand forward, palm facing up, and draw tiny circles in the air with your trusty thumb. Slowly grow those circles to feel more at ease. One direction for 10-15 seconds, then switch for another round.

Tips:

- Keep those fingers and hand chillaxed, focusing on those circular moves.

- Smooth and steady circles, no sudden jolts!

- Any discomfort? Shrink those circles or chat with a healthcare pro.

Thumb circles are a hit in your daily hand workout! Boost thumb mobility and finesse your motor skills. A real lifesaver for managing thumb arthritis, soothing discomfort while keeping those thumbs going strong!

Exercise 8: Hand Spreads

Time to stretch and spread that hand's wings! Start with fingers together and comfy apart. Spread them wide like a bold "V" shape. Hold that stretch for a moment, feeling the hand and fingers stretching like a cat. Bring them back together, open-close, and repeat the smooth moves.

Tips:

- Mindful hand spreads; let the stretch flow through your hand.

- Keep your wrist cool and neutral; no strain here!

- Any woes? Lower the stretch or get pro advice.

Hand spreads are an independence boost! Flex those hands and promote finger independence. Shake off stiffness and unleash your hand's full mobility, just what you need for managing hand osteoarthritis and rocking those daily activities!

Exercise 9: Finger Lifts

Finger lifts are finger-lickin' good! Stretch your hand comfortably, keeping those fingers in line. Starting with the index, Lift one finger at a time. Hold for a few moments; feel those muscles engaged. Gently lower back to the crew, then move on to the middle, ring, and pinky fingers.

Tips:

- Slow and precise finger lifts, one finger at a time, folks.

- Keep your wrist neutral. No stress!

- Any hassle? Lighten the lift or ask a pro.

Finger lifts are the secret to finger strength and control! Give your fingers some TLC, boost their dexterity, and be the master of hand functionality. A real hand-saver for managing hand osteoarthritis and acing your daily deeds!

Exercise 10: Wrist Rolls

Time for wrist rolls; roll it up! Stretch that arm forward, palm up, and gently roll your wrist. Feel the grace in the underside of your arm and wrist. Take 15-30 seconds to savor the stretch. Breathe and feel the release. Swap directions, repeat the serenade on the other hand.

Tips:

- Stay relaxed; let the wrist flow with ease.

- Smooth and gentle rolls, no rush!

- Any trouble? Lighten up or talk to a healthcare pro.

Wrist rolls are a soothing dance for your wrist and forearm. Flexibility and tension relief in one go! An awesome add-on for your hand osteoarthritis management. Kiss stiffness goodbye and savor the wrist's fantastic freedom!

Keep rocking those hand exercises; your fingers will be finger-snapping amazing! Managing osteoarthritis is a breeze when you have these moves in your pocket. Let those hands lead the way to strength and mobility!

Exercise 11: Finger Pinches

Finger pinches are beneficial exercises for hand and finger strength. They can help improve pinch grip and finger coordination, making them valuable for individuals with hand arthritis.

Instructions:

1. Start with your hand comfortably open fingers extended.

2. Gently bring your thumb and index finger together to create a pinch grip.

3. Hold the pinch for a few seconds.

4. Release the pinch and return your fingers to the extended position.

5. Repeat the pinch with your thumb and each of the other fingers in succession.

Tips:

- Perform finger pinches slowly and precisely, focusing on the pinch grip.

- Keep your wrist in a neutral position to avoid strain.

- If you experience any discomfort or pain, reduce the intensity of the pinch or consult a healthcare professional.

Incorporating finger pinches into your daily hand exercise routine can improve hand and finger strength, promoting better grip and dexterity. This exercise is particularly helpful for individuals managing hand arthritis, as it supports hand functionality for various activities throughout the day.

Exercise 12: Hand Grips

Hand grips are strengthening exercises that target your hand and forearm muscles. They can help improve hand grip strength, making them beneficial for individuals with hand osteoarthritis who may experience weakness in their hands.

Instructions:

1. Begin by holding a hand gripper or a soft stress ball in your hand.

2. Squeeze the hand gripper or ball as tightly as you comfortably can.

3. Hold the squeeze for a few seconds.

4. Gradually release the grip and relax your hand.

5. Repeat the squeezing motion 10-15 times with each hand.

Tips:

- Perform hand grips with steady and controlled movements, focusing on the strength of your grip.

- Keep your wrist in a comfortable and neutral position during the exercise.

- If you experience any discomfort or pain, reduce the intensity of the grip or consult a healthcare professional.

Incorporating hand grips into your daily routine can help build hand and forearm strength, making everyday tasks easier and more manageable. This exercise is an excellent addition to your hand osteoarthritis management, enhancing overall hand functionality and grip abilities.

Exercise 13: Thumb Opposition

Thumb opposition is a targeted exercise that aims to improve thumb mobility and coordination. This exercise specifically focuses on the opposition movement of the thumb, which is essential for various fine motor tasks.

Instructions:

1. Start by extending your hand comfortably in front of you with your palm facing upwards.

2. Gently touch your thumb to the base of each finger, one at a time.

3. Begin with your index finger, then move on to your middle finger, ring finger, and pinky finger.

4. After touching each finger, reverse the order and touch your thumb to each finger's base again.

5. Repeat this opposition movement for 10-15 seconds in each direction.

Tips:

- Perform thumb opposition slowly and precisely, focusing on the movement and touch sensation.

- Keep your wrist relaxed and in a neutral position during the exercise.

- If you experience any discomfort or pain, reduce the intensity of the touch or consult a healthcare professional.

Incorporating thumb opposition into your daily hand exercise routine can enhance thumb mobility and fine motor skills. This exercise is particularly beneficial for individuals managing osteoarthritis in the thumb, as it supports overall hand functionality and dexterity.

Exercise 14: Finger Stretch and Curl

Finger stretch and curl is a gentle yet effective exercise that targets finger flexibility and range of motion. This exercise helps to reduce finger stiffness and enhances overall hand mobility, making it beneficial for individuals with hand arthritis.

Instructions:

1. Begin by extending your hand comfortably with your fingers straight.

2. Slowly curl your fingers inward, forming a gentle fist.

3. Hold the fist position for a few seconds, feeling the stretch in your fingers.

4. Gradually release your fingers, straightening them back to their extended position.

5. Repeat this stretching and curling motion 10-15 times.

Tips:

- Perform finger stretch and curl with controlled movements, focusing on the stretch and curl sensation.

- Keep your wrist in a neutral position during the exercise to avoid strain.

- If you experience any discomfort or pain, reduce the intensity of the stretch or consult a healthcare professional.

Incorporating finger stretch and curl into your daily hand exercise routine can maintain finger flexibility and reduce finger stiffness. This exercise is an excellent addition to your hand osteoarthritis management, promoting better hand function for various daily activities.

Exercise 15: Finger Fan-Outs

Finger fan-outs are a good exercise for finger control and independence. It helps improve the coordination of individual finger movements, making it valuable for people with hand arthritis.

Instructions:

1. Start by extending your hand comfortably with your fingers together.

2. Slowly spread your fingers apart as far as you can, creating a fan-like shape with your hand.

3. Hold the fan-out position for a few seconds, feeling the stretch in your fingers.

4. Gradually bring your fingers back together to their original position.

5. Repeat this motion, opening and closing your fingers in a controlled manner.

Tips:

- Do finger fan-outs slowly and precisely, focusing on the movement and spread of your fingers.

- Keep your wrist in a neutral position during the exercise to avoid strain.

- If you feel any discomfort or pain, reduce the intensity of the fan-out or consult a healthcare professional.

You can improve finger coordination and independence by doing finger fan-outs regularly in your hand exercise routine. This exercise is especially helpful for people managing hand arthritis, as it supports hand functionality and enhances fine motor skills for various activities throughout the day.

Congratulations on completing Part Two of our book, where we explored a range of hand exercises designed to alleviate osteoarthritis symptoms and enhance hand health. By incorporating these exercises into your daily routine, you have taken an important step toward improving hand mobility, strength, and flexibility.

Bonus One

Herbal Remedies for Hand Osteoarthritis

Many osteoarthritis patients seek relief from their symptoms through natural herbal remedies and botanical methods. These natural alternatives have proven to be a silent messiah when it comes to osteoarthritis management, and they often go unnoticed. There are many herbs and similar substances that have shown some promise in treating the symptoms of osteoarthritis, let's delve into seven herbs renowned for their promising benefits in handling hand osteoarthritis. Let's discover how to use them, their diverse forms, and where to find them.

Herb 1: Turmeric (Curcuma longa)

Behold the vibrant yellow spice, turmeric, boasting curcumin, a bioactive compound celebrated for its potent anti-inflammatory and antioxidant prowess. This dynamic duo works wonders by diminishing inflammation in afflicted joints and assuaging the discomfort that accompanies hand osteoarthritis.

How to Use

- **Fresh Turmeric:** Grate this golden gem to infuse curries, stews, or smoothies with its magic.

- **Turmeric Powder:** Sprinkle it atop cooked dishes, salads, or indulge in a cup of soothing turmeric-infused milk or tea.

- **Turmeric Supplements:** Available as capsules or tablets; adhere to the recommended dosage on the product label.

Where to Find

- **Fresh Turmeric:** Unearth this treasure trove in most grocery stores flaunting their fresh produce.

- **Turmeric Powder and Supplements:** Seek them out in health food stores and online emporiums.

Herb 2: Ginger (Zingiber officinale)

Step into the warm and spicy realm of ginger, housing gingerols, those dazzling compounds that boast anti-inflammatory prowess. Ginger is on a mission to tame the pain and swelling that's tagged along with hand osteoarthritis.

How to Use

- **Fresh Ginger:** Slice, grate, or mince it to sprinkle culinary charm on dishes, blend it into smoothies, or relish ginger tea's tender embrace after steeping a few slices in hot water for 10 minutes.

- **Ginger Supplements:** Capture ginger's magic in capsules or tablets and follow the recommended dosage to unlock its full potential.

Where to Find

- **Fresh Ginger:** It graces the shelves of most grocery stores.

- **Ginger Supplements:** Seek them out in health food stores and online treasure troves.

Herb 3: Boswellia (Boswellia serrata)

Enter the world of Boswellia, the revered Indian frankincense, bearing boswellic acids as its prized possessions. These valiant acids wield anti-inflammatory powers, endeavoring to curb joint pain and swelling afflicting those grappling with hand osteoarthritis.

How to Use

- **Boswellia Supplements**: Reap the benefits of Boswellia's valor by partaking in capsules or tablets, following the recommended dosage to set sail on the path of relief.

Where to Find

- **Boswellia Supplements:** Chart your course to health food stores and online havens dedicated to herbal treasures.

Herb 4: Devil's Claw (Harpagophytum procumbens)

From the heart of southern Africa springs Devil's Claw, a seasoned herb renowned for easing joint pain. Embrace its active compounds, the heroic harpagosides, stepping forth to showcase their anti-inflammatory prowess.

How to Use

- **Devil's Claw Tea:** Infuse 1 to 2 teaspoons of dried Devil's Claw root in hot water for 10 to 15 minutes, allowing it to unleash its powers.

- **Devil's Claw Supplements:** Enlist the aid of capsules or tablets, following the recommended dosage to tap into Devil's Claw's might.

Where to Find

- **Devil's Claw Products:** Seek refuge in health food stores and virtual marketplaces where treasures abound.

Herb 5: Willow Bark (Salix spp.)

Embark on a journey to discover willow bark, a haven of salicin, nature's counterpart to aspirin, showcasing pain-relieving and anti-inflammatory mastery.

How to Use

- **Willow Bark Tea:** Brew 1 to 2 teaspoons of dried willow bark in hot water for 15 to 20 minutes, unveiling its soothing powers.

- **Willow Bark Supplements:** Engage in capsules or tablets, heeding the recommended dosage to savor its full potential.

Where to Find

- **Willow Bark Products:** Set your course to health food stores and digital bazaars teeming with natural wonders.

Herb 6: Cayenne Pepper (Capsicum annuum)

Ignite your senses with the fiery charm of cayenne pepper, where capsaicin reigns supreme, celebrated for its analgesic might. Unleash its power through topical creams or ointments, tenderly applied to hands ailing from osteoarthritis.

How to Use:

- Cayenne Pepper Spice: Sprinkle the enchanting powder over various dishes, infusing them with its captivating zest.

- Capsaicin Creams: Embrace the gentle touch of topical creams, deftly following the instructions on the label.

Where to Find

- **Cayenne Pepper Spice:** Discover its fiery essence in most grocery stores, tickling taste buds everywhere.

- **Capsaicin Creams:** Uncover these soothing creams in pharmacies and virtual emporiums.

Herb 7: Cat's Claw (Uncaria tomentosa)

Venture into the realm of Cat's Claw, an esteemed herb with a legacy of anti-inflammatory enchantment. Behold the pentacyclic oxindole alkaloids (POAs), poised to relieve joint pain and elevate hand osteoarthritis well-being.

How to Use:

- Cat's Claw Supplements: Embrace the allure of capsules or tablets, heeding the recommended dosage to traverse the path of relief.

Where to Find:

- Cat's Claw Supplements: Set your sights on health food stores and digital sanctuaries teeming with herbal wonders.

Enrich your daily routine with the seven herbal champions - turmeric, ginger, boswellia, devil's claw, willow bark, cayenne pepper, and cat's claw - as allies in your battle against hand osteoarthritis. Nevertheless, remember that these herbal remedies complement, but do not replace, medical advice and care. Consult a healthcare professional, especially if you have underlying health conditions, allergies, or are taking medications that may interact with these remedies.

These herbal treasures can be found in a diverse array of locales, from grocery store shelves to health food stores, and virtual marketplaces brimming with herbal wisdom. Make discerning choices, ensuring quality and potency. By combining these natural marvels with anti-inflammatory diet, exercise, and lifestyle adaptations, you can navigate hand osteoarthritis with renewed vigor and embrace improved well-being.

Bonus Two

Hot and Cold Therapy for Osteoarthritis Relief

Hot and cold therapy, two powerful methods to alleviate hand osteoarthritis bring relief through their unique applications of heat and cold. These therapeutic approaches offer diverse benefits to ease pain and inflammation, providing a soothing warmth or numbing chill to the affected hands. When it comes to managing osteoarthritis discomfort, hot and cold therapy prove to be simple yet potent allies.

Why Consider Using Hot and Cold Therapy for Hands with Osteoarthritis?

1. **Natural Pain Relief**: Embracing the simplicity of hot and cold therapy means embracing a drug-free path to soothe hand osteoarthritis pain. With these techniques, individuals can rely less on medications and embrace more natural relief.

2. **Reduction of Inflammation:** Hot and cold therapy take different routes to tackle inflammation. Heat turns up the blood flow to the area, promoting healing and melting stiffness away. In contrast, cold therapy chills out the blood vessels, fighting off swelling and numbing the discomfort.

3. **Enhanced Hand Mobility:** As pain recedes and inflammation subsides, hand mobility and flexibility experience a rejuvenating boost with hot and cold therapy. Everyday tasks become smoother, more manageable, and more enjoyable.

4. **Non-Invasive and Safe:** There's no need to invade or risk when using hot and cold therapy. These gentle methods can be comfortably administered at home, putting individuals in control of their arthritis treatment.

5. **Cost-Effective:** When comparing costs, hot and cold therapy triumph as cost-effective warriors. Reusable ice packs and heating pads won't burn holes in wallets, making them budget-friendly alternatives.

6. **Personalized Approach:** Hand osteoarthritis is a unique journey for each individual, and hot and cold therapy readily adapt to cater to personal preferences. The therapies offer an open canvas for experimentation, allowing patients to discover what works best for their distinctive symptoms.

7. **Convenient and Accessible:** Hot and cold therapy blend seamlessly into daily routines, creating accessible options for quick relief. A morning warm soak or an after-activity cold compress grants easy access to the therapeutic benefits.

Cold Therapy for Soothing Hand Osteoarthritis Pain

Enter the realm of cryotherapy, where cold therapy emerges as a wondrous ally, easing hand osteoarthritis pain and quelling inflammation.

Getting Started

1. **Consult with Your Healthcare Provider:** Before venturing into the frosty embrace of cold therapy, seek the

counsel of your healthcare provider. Let their wisdom shine, offering personalized advice for your unique situation.

2. **Select the Cold Source:** An array of options beckon—ice packs, frozen gel packs, even frozen veggies nestled in a gentle cloth. Choose the companion that caresses your hand with tender chill and convenience.

3. **Create a Relaxing Environment:** Create a sanctuary of serenity where cold therapy thrives, free from worldly distractions. Keep your cold source close, and perhaps a timer to mark the cadence of your therapy.

How to Perform Cold Therapy

1. **Prepare the Cold Source:** Prepare your ice pack or gel pack as instructed, chilling it to the perfect temperature. For frozen veggies, swaddle them tenderly in a thin cloth or towel.

2. **Wrap the Cold Source:** Shield your skin from the icy touch, wrapping the cold source in a gentle cloth or towel. Frostbite shall be thwarted, your skin untouched.

3. **Apply to the Affected Area:** Gently lay the wrapped cold source upon your painful or swollen hand, bestowing its comforting chill with grace and precision.

4. **Duration of Therapy:** Abide by the siren's call—10 to 15 minutes per session, the golden rule for this cold ballet. Do not linger beyond this limit, lest the skin gods frown.

5. **Frequency of Use:** For more icy respite, indulge in multiple cold therapy sessions daily, mindful not to court frostbite. Grant your skin intervals of warmth between each rendezvous.

Safety Guidelines

1. **Avoid Direct Contact:** Pledge to keep the cold source from directly touching your skin, enshrouding it in a tender cloth or towel. Frostbite's advances shall be thwarted.

2. **Monitor Your Skin:** Keep watchful eyes upon your skin, vigilant for signs of redness or numbness. If peril appears, discontinue the therapy at once.

3. **Not Suitable for Everyone:** Bear in mind that cold therapy may spurn those with certain medical conditions like Raynaud's disease. Consult your healthcare provider before embarking on this chilly quest.

4. **Combine with Other Treatments:** Unveil the secret of synergy by coupling cold therapy with other treatments, like hand exercises or the medicines bestowed upon you by your healthcare provider.

5. **Avoid on Open Wounds:** A solemn edict—cold therapy shall not grace open wounds or broken skin. Obey this command to fend off the specter of infection.

Cold therapy stands poised, ready to release your hand from the clutches of osteoarthritis pain and inflammation. With technique and safety as your guides, embark on this journey of simple and effective treatment. Seek professional guidance before welcoming new treatments to your arthritis management plan, and witness a golden future of hand health and well-being.

Hot Therapy to Soothe Hand Osteoarthritis

Prepare to enter a realm of solace and healing, where the magic of hot therapy awaits, a comforting elixir for hand osteoarthritis. Envelop yourself in the tender embrace of warmth and embark on a divine journey of relief. To embark on this enchanting path, arm yourself with the essentials and follow the beguiling steps that weave the spell of hot therapy.

Essentials materials you will need

1. **Heating Pad or Warm Compress:** Revel in the company of a faithful companion - a reliable heating pad or warm compress. Let the magic of heat unfold before you, caressing your hand with a gentle warmth, coaxing away the cold clutches of osteoarthritis.

2. **Towel or Cloth:** Adorn your chosen ally, the heating pad or warm compress, with a soft and cozy towel or cloth, a guardian against skin sensitivity. For in the mystical realm of hot therapy, the well-being of your delicate skin reigns supreme.

3. **Find Serenity in a Relaxing Space:** Seek refuge in a sanctuary of serenity, where the enchanting spell of hot therapy can weave undisturbed. Create a haven of peace, where the mystical magic shall unfold its wondrous tapestry.

How to Perform Hot Therapy

1. **Prepare the Warming Embrace:** Awaken the magic by preparing your chosen ally, the heating pad or warm compress, embracing it with a cozy and comfortable temperature. Witness the spell of heat being woven, as it soothes and calms your afflicted hand.

2. **Wrap in the Tender Embrace:** With tender care, cradle your heating pad or warm compress in the loving cocoon of a soft and cozy cloth. Safeguard your skin from the intensity

of direct contact, for in the realm of hot therapy, gentleness holds the key.

3. **Nestle in Comfort**: Seek a state of pure comfort, nestling your hand upon the welcoming warmth. Feel the tender heat enveloping your hand, casting aside tensions and inviting tranquility.

4. **Savor the Enchanting Warmth**: Allow time to become your ally, savoring the comforting warmth as it works its enchantment on your hand. Inhale serenity as the nurturing heat weaves its healing touch upon your hand.

5. **Embrace the Magic for 15-20 Minutes**: Rejoice in the spellbinding magic of hot therapy for a sacred window of 15-20 minutes per session. Within this enchanted timeframe, the gentle heat weaves its wonders, comforting your hand with grace.

6. **The Allure of Frequency**: Embrace the allure of hot therapy 2-3 times a day, guided by the whispers of your hand

osteoarthritis needs. Allow the tenderness of the warmth to linger, as it works its magic to relieve your discomfort.

7. Farewell with Gratitude: As each session concludes, bid farewell to the warm embrace, grateful for the relief it bestowed. Rest assured, the comforting touch shall be summoned again whenever needed.

Safety Guidelines

1. Guard your hand from undue harm, cloaking the heating pad or warm compress in the gentle embrace of a soft cloth before applying to your skin.

2. Honor the boundaries of time, allowing hot therapy sessions to last no longer than 20 minutes, a safeguard against potential skin sensitivity.

In this wondrous realm of hot therapy, the tender warmth heals and nurtures, offering a journey of healing and relief for your hand osteoarthritis. Embark on this beguiling path, and let the enchantment unfold with every touch, as your hand rejoices in the embrace of healing warmth.

Conclusion

In this comprehensive book, we have explored a holistic approach to hand health, including exercises designed to reduce osteoarthritis symptoms and improve overall hand well-being. Additionally, we have provided valuable insight into anti-inflammatory recipes, a 7-day meal plan, and bonus herbal recipes to add to your workout routine

Through a journey of knowledge and understanding, we have empowered readers with practical and effective techniques to improve hand movement, strength and flexibility. Exercises that are optimized for convenience and effectiveness have the potential to make a huge difference in the lives of individuals managing chiropractic care

Additionally, our bonus herbal treatment offers a natural complement to traditional treatments, as well as the hot and cold therapy. These innovative solutions have the potential to provide additional relief and enhance overall well-being.

As our journey draws to a close, let's celebrate the progress we've made and the small victories we've celebrated. Knowledge gained here will be a powerful tool in the pursuit of increased handedness and pain relief.

Armed with this new knowledge, it is our sincere hope that readers will engage in a lifelong commitment to hand health. By embracing exercise and nutrient-dense cooking, we invite everyone to unlock the power of their hands and enrich their lives with improved mobility and reduced harm.

A heartfelt thank you to every reader who has traveled with us on this transformative journey. Together, we embrace the power of hands-on exercises, healthy food, and the gift of natural herbs. Let this comprehensive guide be a definite companion on the road to a healthy and happy life

Appreciation

We want to express our heartfelt gratitude to each and every reader who has chosen to embark on this journey with us through ***"Healing Osteoarthritis Hands"***

Your trust in our book is a true honor, and we are humbled by the opportunity to be a part of your experience.

We encourage you to make the most of our book by utilizing our free consultation via email wintonconsults@gmail.com We are here to listen, support, and provide guidance as you navigate the challenges osteoarthritis. Bear in mind that your personal experiences and challenges are valuable, and by sharing them, you can inspire and encourage others who may be facing similar difficulties.

As a show of appreciation, we humbly ask for your ratings and kind review using our book.

Together, let's create a community where we uplift and empower one another. We are committed to your well-being and the well-being of your hands.

Yours Sincerely,

DR. KADEN WINTON & TEAM.

Picture Links

https://images.pexels.com/photos/54321/hand-elderly-woman-wrinkles-black-and-white-54321.jpeg?auto=compress&cs=tinysrgb&w=1260&h=750&dpr=1

https://www.pexels.com/photo/persons-left-hand-4061223/

https://images.pexels.com/photos/7298394/pexels-photo-7298394.jpeg?auto=compress&cs=tinysrgb&w=600

https://www.pexels.com/photo/close-up-shot-of-a-stretching-hands-7298387/

https://images.pexels.com/photos/6888687/pexels-photo-6888687.jpeg?auto=compress&cs=tinysrgb&w=600&lazy=load

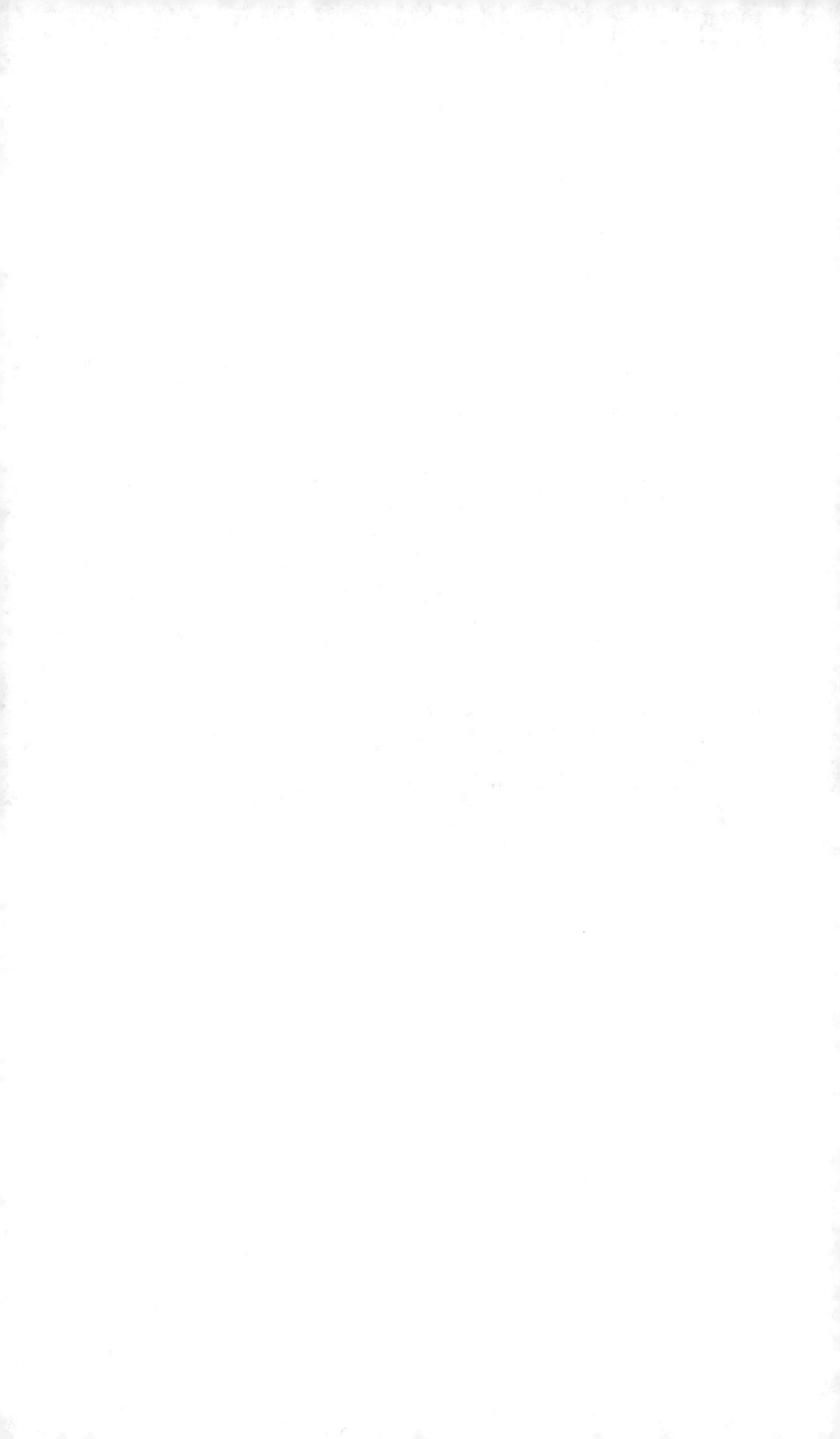